Ting-Kai Leung
Shoei-Loong Lin

MRI explains herbal estrogen increase breast cancer risk or prevention

Ting-Kai Leung
Shoei-Loong Lin

MRI explains herbal estrogen increase breast cancer risk or prevention

Breast MRI characteristics under hormone effects and epidemiology of breast cancer in Taiwan

LAP LAMBERT Academic Publishing

Impressum / Imprint

Bibliografische Information der Deutschen Nationalbibliothek: Die Deutsche Nationalbibliothek verzeichnet diese Publikation in der Deutschen Nationalbibliografie; detaillierte bibliografische Daten sind im Internet über http://dnb.d-nb.de abrufbar.

Alle in diesem Buch genannten Marken und Produktnamen unterliegen warenzeichen-, marken- oder patentrechtlichem Schutz bzw. sind Warenzeichen oder eingetragene Warenzeichen der jeweiligen Inhaber. Die Wiedergabe von Marken, Produktnamen, Gebrauchsnamen, Handelsnamen, Warenbezeichnungen u.s.w. in diesem Werk berechtigt auch ohne besondere Kennzeichnung nicht zu der Annahme, dass solche Namen im Sinne der Warenzeichen- und Markenschutzgesetzgebung als frei zu betrachten wären und daher von jedermann benutzt werden dürften.

Bibliographic information published by the Deutsche Nationalbibliothek: The Deutsche Nationalbibliothek lists this publication in the Deutsche Nationalbibliografie; detailed bibliographic data are available in the Internet at http://dnb.d-nb.de.

Any brand names and product names mentioned in this book are subject to trademark, brand or patent protection and are trademarks or registered trademarks of their respective holders. The use of brand names, product names, common names, trade names, product descriptions etc. even without a particular marking in this works is in no way to be construed to mean that such names may be regarded as unrestricted in respect of trademark and brand protection legislation and could thus be used by anyone.

Coverbild / Cover image: www.ingimage.com

Verlag / Publisher:
LAP LAMBERT Academic Publishing
ist ein Imprint der / is a trademark of
OmniScriptum GmbH & Co. KG
Heinrich-Böcking-Str. 6-8, 66121 Saarbrücken, Deutschland / Germany
Email: info@lap-publishing.com

Herstellung: siehe letzte Seite /
Printed at: see last page
ISBN: 978-3-659-49175-7

MRI explains herbal estrogen increase breast cancer risk or prevention

Ting-Kai Leung, MD(Ass.Professor of Radiology)   Shoei-Loong Lin,MD(Clinical Professor of Surgery)

Table of Contents

Incidence of breast cancer in Taiwan

Breast cancer is one of the most common cancers and is the leading cause of

cancer-related death in women throughout the world. Over the past two decades in

Taiwan, the incidence of breast cancer is increasing. It was also found a sharp rise

of breast cancer mortality and shows no sign of slowing down. In most of the

public believe, this increase may be caused by changes in lifestyle, into more

Westernization.

On the other hand, the mean age of Taiwanese breast cancer patients are often

younger than Western countries[1,2]. In Taiwan, about 50% of the newly clinical

diagnosis of breast cancer cases occur in patients of 45-50 year old. In contrast, in

Western countries, the majority of newly diagnosed breast cancer patients are over

50 years old in United States[1]. In addition, the equivalent peak of Taiwanese

occurred 5 to 10 years younger that United States. And it was found the younger

age of less than 45 years old female breast cancer women were increasing rapidly

in Taiwan[1,2,3].

3

Interestingly, the prevalence of breast cancer is lower in Taiwanese (ethnic Chinese)

populations than in Caucasian populations, and the epidemiological patterns are

different in the two patient groups. First, the median age of breast cancer patients in

Taiwan (45–49 years) is lesser than that in Western countries (70–74 years). Second,

a rise in incidence has been observed consistently in Asian countries [4,5,6], and

one age-period-cohort analysis showed that the increase in breast cancer incidence

was largely due to a rise in young patients. Third, it was revealed that young breast

cancer patients in Taiwan carried a greater risk and shorter interval progression than

in western women[7,8]. As the young age and bilateral breast cancer are more

likely to be related to genetic predisposal of factors [9,10], it is important to

identify potential predisposing factors in Taiwanese patients.

Genetic factors

According to our clinical observation, family factor with having a mother or sister

diagnosed with breast cancer, is the highest risk of breast cancer to other female

members. Unlike Western countries, such as United States, the precise genetic risk

calculation on the probability of breast cancer of the individual woman with

positive history is still not clear. Although evidence suggests an importance of

genetic factors in the development of breast cancer in Taiwanese (ethnic Chinese)

women, including a high incidence of early-onset and secondary contralateral

4

breast cancer, a major breast cancer predisposition gene, BRCA1, has not been well

studied in this population. In fact, the carcinogenic impacts of many genetic

variants of BRCA1

are unknown and classified as variants of uncertain significance in most of

Asian-Pacific countries. Although several studies detected the BRCA1 germ-line

mutations in Chinese women with familial breast cancer, most of them did not

employ conventional full gene sequencing[11]. Only small scale studies were

performed in Taiwan, as well as other Asian-Pacific countries. A previous study

found 27.7%(5/18) of the families with multiple cases of Taiwanese breast

cancer ,were found to carry cancer-associated gene mutations in the BRCA1 and

BRCA2 genes. Several genetic polymorphisms in both BRCA1 and BRCA2 genes

were also detected in this investigation[12]. Immunohistochemistry analyses were

performed on tumor samples to detect the expression of estrogen receptor (ER),

progesterone receptor (PR), P53, and human epidermal growth factor receptor-2

(HER-2). Asian breast cancer patients having one or more affected relatives, minor

study was found BRCA1 germ-line mutation rate at 11.3% (gene2). BRCA1

mutation tumors tended to be negative for ER, PR, and HER-2, and exhibited high

histological grade compared with tumors without BRCA1 mutations[13]. The

BRCA1 and BRCA2 genes are the strongest susceptibility genes identified for breast cancer worldwide. However, BRCA1/BRCA2 have been incompletely

investigated due to their large size and the genomic rearrangements that

occasionally occur within them. It was performed a comprehensive mutational

analysis for BRCA1/BRCA2 in 206 Korean patients with breast cancer. From the

results, 38 patients (18.4%) had one or more BRCA1/BRCA2 mutations. No large

deletions or duplications involving BRCA1/BRCA2 were identified.

BRCA1/BRCA2 mutations were more frequent in a group with family history,

bilateral cancer or multiple site cancer than in a group without the risk factors

described or an unknown risk group. Mutation frequencies in the early-onset cancer

group were not higher than in the unknown risk group[14].On the contrary,

according to a large population based study in Britain, the prevalence of BRCA1

and BRCA2 mutations was found in 11% of patients with a first-degree relative

who developed ovarian cancer or breast cancer by age 60 years. And, the

percentage elevated to 45% of patients with two or more affected first- or

second-degree relatives mutation carriers[15]. Genetic factors related to breast

cancer, including BRCA1, have not been well studied in the Asia-Pacific

areas(gene1-4). Although several studies detected the BRCA1 germ-line mutations

in Taiwanese women with familial breast cancer, most of them did not employ

conventional full gene sequencing. In addition, breast cancer predisposition genes identified, such as BRCA1 and BRCA2, are found responsible for less than 5% of

all breast cancer cases[16]. In Taiwan, past studies found a few benign

polymorphisms of BRCA1 without the identification of pathological mutants

associated with breast cancer development[17,18].Without strong relationship on

most of Taiwanese breast cancer patients on genetic factor, there were only gene

deletion or frame-shift mutation of the BRCA1 gene could be clearly defined as a

deleterious mutant (gene1). Past studies in Taiwan, found a few benign

polymorphisms of BRCA1 without the identification of pathological mutants

associated with breast cancer development[17,18]. There were only gene deletion

or frame-shift mutation of the BRCA1 gene could be clearly defined as a

deleterious mutant[11]. Of the reported studies conducted in other Asian-Pacific

countries, such as China, Korea, Japan and Malaysia, germ-line BRCA1 mutation

occurred in approximately 4–9% of breast cancer patients[19,20,21,22].This is

lower than the ~10% reported in non-Jewish Caucasian women with early-onset or

a familial history of breast cancer.

Estrogen factor

In Western countries, hormone replacement therapy (HRT) is believed or regarded as

one of the major risk factor for breast cancer. Since 2000 , the application of HRT

in Germany, was significantly reduction in the total population. In the meanwhile, the incidence of breast cancer is coincidence decline in 2000 and 2005[23]. This finding should be interpretation as a positive relationship between HRT and breast cancer.

Taiwanese breast cancer in premenopausal women, the incidence is higher; reflecting in breast cancer and estrogen supplements may have a specific relationship pattern. Previous experiments indicated that estrogens promote the development of mammary cancer in rodents and exert both direct and indirect proliferative effects on cultured breast-cancer cells from humans[24].

Direct tumor-initiating effects may occur through the induction of enzymes and proteins involved in nucleic acid synthesis and through the activation of oncogenes. Indirect effects may occur through the stimulation of prolactin secretion and the production of growth factors (e.g., transforming growth factor α and epidermal growth factor) and non–growth-factor peptides (e.g., plasminogen activators). Tumor formation may also result from excessive hormonal stimulation of an organ in which normal growth and function are under endocrine control[25]. The response of an organ to the proliferative effects of a hormone may be a progression from normal growth to hyperplasia to neoplasm. In this model, the risk of breast cancer could be determined by the cumulative exposure of breast tissue to estrogen [26]. Indirect evidence of this sequence includes the increased risk of breast cancer associated with early menstruation, late first full-term pregnancy, late menopausal

and reduced risk associated with early menopause[27,28].

Genetic and environmental factors influence estrogen homeostasis and tissue-specific

exposure to estrogen and its metabolites. The relative influence of the fluctuating

serum estrogen concentrations associated with the menstrual cycle in

premenopausal women and the more stable concentrations in postmenopausal

women on the cumulative lifetime exposure to estrogen is uncertain. Taken together,

the body of data supports the hypothesis that estrogen and its metabolites are

related to both the initiation and the promotion of breast cancer but that these

associations are complicated [29].

Estrogen-like Herb and the related Herb Supplements

Many herbs were traditionally used by herbalists for treating a variety of health

problems were extracted and tested for their relative capacity to compete with

estradiol and progesterone binding to intracellular receptors for progesterone (PR)

and estradiol (ER) in intact human breast cancer cells. The ones possessing high

ER-binding herbs that are commonly consumed were soy, licorice, red clover,

thyme, tumeric, hops, and verbena. The ones possessing high PR-binding herbs and

spices commonly consumed were oregano, verbena, tumeric, thyme, red clover and

damiana. Some of the herbs and spices found to contain high phytoestrogens (genistein (genistein), evening primrose oil, yam extract (yam extract) and royal jelly); or phytoprogestins were further tested for bioactivity based on their ability to regulate cell growth rate in ER (+) and ER (-) breast cancer cell lines and to induce or inhibit the synthesis of alkaline phosphatase, an end product of progesterone action, in PR (+) cells. Basically, ER-binding herbal extracts were agonists, the ER stimulate effect similar to estradiol. On the other hand, PR-binding extracts, were neutral or antagonists. In vivo, the bioavailability of phytoestrogens and phytoprogestins were quantitatively studied on the ER-binding and PR-binding capacity of saliva following consumption of soy milk, it was found soy milk exhibits a dramatic increase in saliva ER-binding components. After consumption of PR-binding herbs(exogenous progesterone, medroxyprogesterone acetate, and wild mexican yam products containing diosgenin), it increased the progestin activity of saliva, but there were significant differences in their individual bioactivity [30,31]. In our opinion, as the rapid developing technologies on herbal extraction and purification, its clinical outcome and pharmacological effect become more advance, it should be more concern on the possible adverse effects on different herbal supplements[32].

Breast glandular cells contain cell membrane receptors for estrogen and other receptors for progesterone. Approximately 3 quarters of all breast cancers are estrogen receptor positive (ER-positive), which means estrogen causes these tumors to grow. However, during malignant transformation, breast cancer cells do not distinguish between estrogen and phytoestrogen ingested by the patient [2,33,34,35].

Synthetic chemical estrogen (such as xenoestrogen) may take months to metabolize and pass out of the patient's body. The use of chemical estrogens has been found to correlate strongly with an increased incidence of breast cancer. In contrast, most food grade estrogen supplements or phytoestrogens are metabolized and pass out of the body in several days to weeks. Thus, short-term use of phytoestrogens may be poorly correlated with breast cancer incidence, but long-term or over-use of the same products may not be safe. Although extracted from plant tissue, phytoestrogen supplements intended to reduce menopausal symptoms may not provide protection from breast cancer [36,37,38]. Studies conducted with human breast cancer cell lines indicate that genistein both inhibits and stimulates proliferation of these cells. A mitogenic effect of genistein was observed at low doses, but an antiproliferative effect at higher doses. The growth of murine breast cancer cell lines with estrogen-positive receptor (MCF-7 cells) was first stimulated and then inhibited by genistein in a dose- dependent manner [39,40,41]. One study found that genistein exerted different effects on the breast depending on the timing of exposure. In addition, hytoestrogen-genistein may interfere with the inhibitive effects of

tamoxifen on breast cancer cell growth [42]. Nevertheless, the potential cancer-

promoting effect of genistein should not be omitted [43]. In Asian regions,

including Mainland China, Taiwan, Hong Kong and Singapore, many women seek

natural supplements or traditional Chinese herbal support for the relief of

menopause symptoms [44]. In the mean while, phytoestrogen extracted from

natural sources or traditional Chinese herbs may stimulate the proliferation of

breast cancer cell line (MCF-7) [43]. Several studies have analyzed the effects of

various herbal supplements and medications. Cell cycle analysis has revealed that

the stimulation of proliferation may be associated with a marked in- crease in the

replication of MCF-7 cells, with the effects being similar to that of human estradiol

[45,46,47,48]. In this book, we introduce the two natural supplement and herb

(geinstein and ginseng), they probably received the mostly applications and

scientific studies around the world, including on pre-menopausal syndrome.

Phytoestrogens are non-steroidal compounds that occur naturally in plants and that

possess weak estrogenic activity [49,50]. Estrogen-like responses have been

reported for chemicals such as flavonoids, coumestans, and stilbenes [49,51]. The

potential biological impact of phytoestrogens has generated considerable interest.

Phytoestrogens interact with nuclear ER through which they could modulate a variety of estrogen-dependent processes. Ginseng has also been a popular herb for

the alleviation of menopausal symptoms. Despite the extensive use of ginseng as an

alternative for hormone replacement therapy, but it is necessary to understand the

molecular mechanisms and efficacy of ginseng for safer use of this promising

alternative therapy[49]

(1)Geinstein

Genistein is a phytoestrogen and belongs to the category of isoflavones. Isoflavones

such as genistein and daidzein are found in a number of plants including lupin, fava

beans, soybeans, kudzu, and psoralea being the primary food source, especially to

many Asian countries. According to the recent studies and scientific researches, it

was found that Genistein or isoflavones have been linked to both beneficial as well

as adverse effects in relation to cell proliferation and cancer risks. It was present an

overview study on isoflavones that it may bearing contradicting health effects, and

of mechanisms that could be conduct dualistic mode of action. One mechanism

relates to the different ultimate cellular effects of activation of estrogen receptor

(ER), promoting cell proliferation(include malignant breast cells), but also

promoting apoptosis of malignant breast cells. The overview was reflected that

scientists are only at the start of unraveling the complex underlying mode of action

for effects of isoflavones, both beneficial or adverse, on cell proliferation and

13

cancer risks(52).In conclusion, short-term dietary soy intake has a weak estrogenic

response on the breast, but without antiestrogenic effect (53).

Prolonged consumption of soy protein isolate has a stimulatory effect on the

premenopausal female breast, characterized by increased secretion of breast fluid,

promote hyperplastic change of epithelial cells, as well as elevate levels of plasma E2.

Nevertheless, it was suggested that soybean isoflavones exert an estrogenic

stimulus on breast tissue [53]. In a recent randomized double blind phase II trial

conducted by Khan et al. [54] examined the effects of 6-month soy isoflavone

supplementation on breast epithelial cell proliferation and other biomarkers,

including gene expression detecting apoptosis, proliferation, and estrogenicity, as

well as hormone levels in the nipple aspirate fluid. In their study, a 6-month

intervention with mixed soy isoflavones in healthy, high-risk adult Western women

did not reduce breast epithelial cell proliferation, suggesting a lack of efficacy for

breast cancer prevention and even possible adverse effects in premenopausal

women, reflected by the increase in the Ki-67 labeling index, which is a marker for

cell proliferation [54]. Given the concerns over the induction or potentiation of

carcinogenesis due to its weak estrogenic activity, genistein was selected by the

National Toxicology Program as one of the compounds to be examined for

long-term adverse effects in a 2-year rat study at different dose levels for diets [55].

It was found soybean exhibits early onset of aberrant estrous cycles, suggesting

early reproductive senescence, and significantly increased pituitary weights were

observed for the high-dose group. There was some evidence of carcinogenic

activity of genistein in female rats based on increased incidences of mammary

gland adenoma or (combined) and pituitary gland neoplasms [55]. A hypothesis put

forward to explain the seemingly contradictory health effects of estrogens and

phytoestrogens relates to the potentially different ultimate cellular effect of

activation activation of ER, promoting cell proliferation and possible adverse health

effects(56-63).

(2) Ginseng

There were several studies on the estrogenic activity of a component of

ginseng(ginsenoside-Rb1)(Gi) [64,65]. Gi activated both estrogen and

progesterone receptor receptors in a dose-dependent manner. Activation was

inhibited by the estrogen receptor antagonist, indicating that the effects were

mediated through the estrogen receptor. Like 17-estradiol, treatment with Gi also

increased expression of the progesterone receptor and estrogen receptor in ER

positive breast cancer cell line(MCF-7 cells) .It was suggest that Gi is functionally

very similar to 17-estradiol in MCF-7 breast cancer cells. The estrogen-like activity

of Gi is independent of direct estrogen receptor association. In conclusion, in-vitro mechanism of Gi leads to ER activation[64]. Gi has been recommended to alleviate

the menopausal symptoms, which indicates that components of ginseng very likely

contain estrogenic activity. Accurately, Gi activated the transcription of the

estrogen-responsive gene receptor in MCF-7 breast cancer cells. Thus, Gi acts a

weak phytoestrogen, presumably by binding and activating the estrogen

receptor[64,65].

Mammographic density and hormone replacement therapy(HRT)

It was already known that elevated mammographic density is strongly associated with

breast cancer risk and the estrogen pathway has been proposed as a potential

mechanism for this association. It has been repeatedly observed that several

established estrogen-related factors associated with breast cancer risk, such as parity

and hormone replacement therapy, are also associated with mammographic density.

However, the association of circulating estrogen levels (known to be strongly

positively associated with breast cancer risk) with mammographic density has so

far been inconsistent. Since mammographic density is highly heritable, the risk

factor on breast cancer with mammographic density is hardly determined. It was

showed no association with mammographic density to hormone effect when

analyses were performed on overall study population. However, when this relation was assessed within strata based on estrogen-related factors, seemed to be related to mammographic density in the same direction of their associations with breast cancer risk. A previous study was emphasis the importance of radiographic image on breast cancer risk, related to bio-molecular and gene factor(mammo1-2). While other studies have shown that use of postmenopausal hormone therapy with estrogen and progestogen increases mammographic density. Mammographic density differed by type of hormone therapy used, dose, duration and whether the effects are modified by age and body mass index (BMI).Under assessed with a computer assisted method, was found higher mammographic density was among current hormone replacement users. The highest density was seen in current therapy with both estrogen and progestogen users who had a average increased percent density of over 26%[66,67].

Breast MRI

MRI for detecting breast lesions is extremely sensitive. It can identify breast cancer at an early stage of the formation of abnormal proliferation, vascular proliferation (angiogenesis) and vascular permeability (microvascular permeability) state.

Our analysis of the patient's breast MRI images, known estrogen and phytoestrogen intake and cancer risk is related to the MRI imaging , we assessed estrogen and phytoestrogens on breast glandular tissue is influential.

Major group(all participants)

We collected from 2008 to 2012, 2795 cases of women who participate in our hospital

MRI imaging examination. This women undergoing MRI examination , the need to

3 days before menstruation or after 7 days between the effects of estrogen in order

to reduce the possibility of imaging results .

Minor group(HRT and phytoestrogen users)

From 2010 to 2012, a total of 219 women in the experimental group was selected

images. These women are doing before the MRI examination , has received at least

three months of estrogen supplements , estrogen ingredients or plant estrogens

(including herbal or Chinese herbs such as genistein (genistein), evening primrose

oil, yam extract (yam extract), fungus, royal jelly) .

BIRADS classification in breast MRI

Breast Imaging Reporting and Data System (BI-RADS), to BRMRI interpreted and

adopted a standard of ACR BIRADS MRI [68,69,70,71,72,73]. Imaging results

BI-RADS score Class 1 or Class 2 refers to the results of normal and benign , there

is no risk of malignancy . If the image is the result score of category 3 (probably

benign) , Type 4 (suspicious abnormality) , category 5 (highly suggestive of

malignancy) , or section 6 (a known malignancy) , these instructions the patient's

cancer risk.

2.5 Health and interpretation of the classification of breast unhealthy

We use a simple classification system , MRI BI-RADS classification level in the

BI-RADS Ⅲ, Ⅳ, Ⅴ, Ⅵ Ⅰ, Ⅱ and "unhealthy" image was named "healthy"

received image .

Statistical healthy and unhealthy Comparison of breast images

Were analyzed using SPSS statistical software . We compared the results of the

binomial test samples for at least three months use of estrogen and phytoestrogens

in the minor group and the major group (study population) . AP value less than

0.05 was considered statistically significant.

Healthy and unhealthy image ratio

Preliminary results of Breast MRI studied on estrogen or phytoestrogen users

We analyzed the results for all 2795 images of women who had received breast MRI

screening at our hospital. We classified 50.86% of the images as healthy (BIRADS

I, II) and unhealthy images accounted for 48.66% (BIRADS III, IV, V, VI) of our

study population. Within the total study group, a subgroup of 219 images of women

had reported taking estrogen or phytoestrogen regularly for at least 3 months. We

retrospectively reviewed their MRI results and classified 34.67% of the breast

images from this subgroup as healthy, thus, 65.33% of the breast images were

classified unhealthy (Figure1). It showed a statistically significant difference ($p <$

0.001), indicating that women taking estrogen or phytoestrogen supplements had a

greater tendency to develop breast disease or unhealthy breast conditions (Table1).

	Healthy breast MRI results (BIRADS I 、 II)	Unhealthy breast MRI results (BIRADS 、 III 、 IV 、 V 、 VI)	P
All women screened (n=2795)	1360	1435	
Estrogen-like group (n=150)	52	98	0.0010***

***Statistically significant at $P < 0.001$.

Table 1. *Comparison of MRI images in the study population and a subgroup of estrogen users.*

20

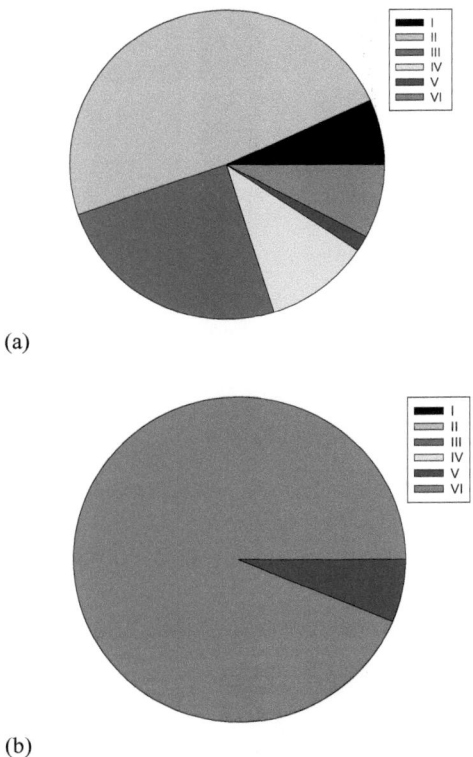

(a)

(b)

Figure 1. *BIRADS grading of the study population (a) and a subgroup of estrogen*

users (b).

Our results also indicated that physiological cycles and natural supplements such as

genistein, royal jelly, evening primrose oil, yam extract, and Ganoderma lucidum

could stimulate breast glandular tissue in the same way as HRT, yielding a positive

proliferative change, detectable on MRI images(Figure2-10).

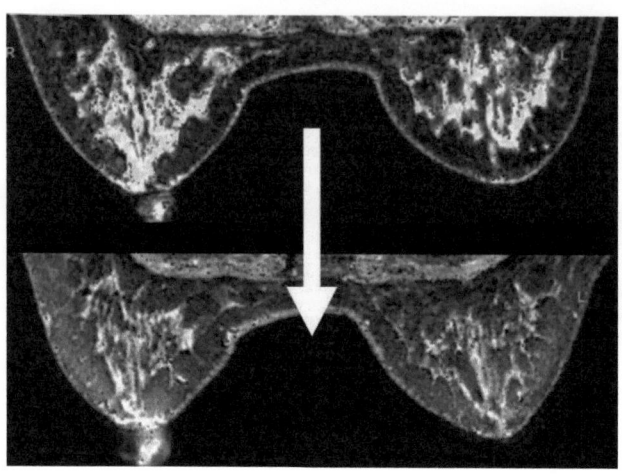

Figure 2 Before menstruation, MRI shows diffusely glandular enhancement of

contrast enhanced dynamic MRI. After 2 years, as menopause, there is significant

regress change without post contrast enhancement of breast glandular tissue.

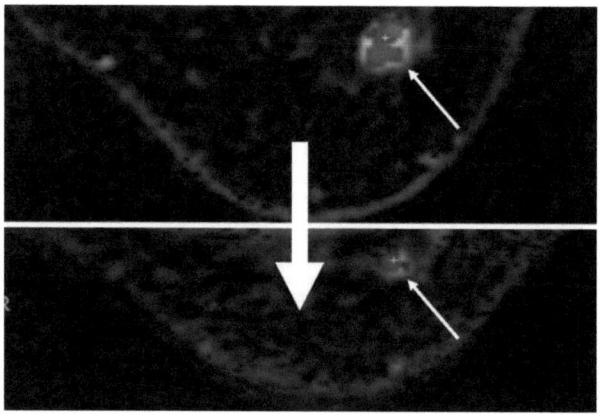

Figure 3 Before menstruation, MRI shows probably benign fibroadenoma at left

breast. Under enhanced dynamic MRI. After 2 years, as menopause, there is

significant regression of previous mentioned fibroadenoma with lesser of enhancement and shrinkage of tumor size.

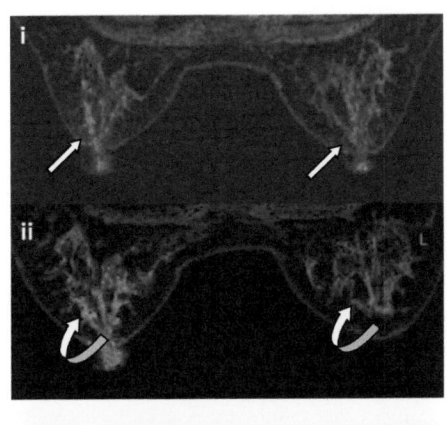

(a)

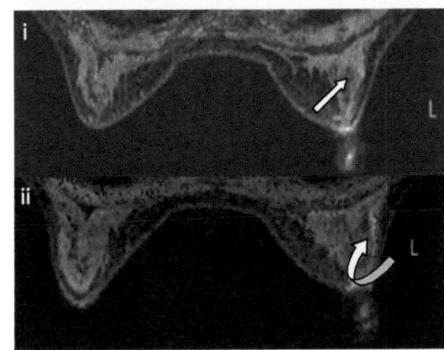

(b)

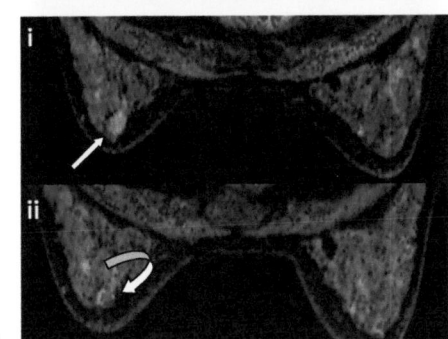

(c)

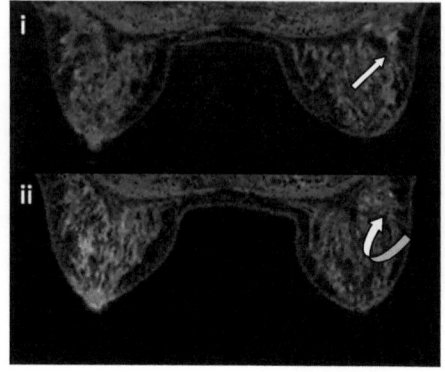

(d)

Figure 4a-4d . *(i) It shows normal signal and color mapping of breast epithelial tissue by breast MRI post-processing (straight arrows); (ii) after estrogen therapy or phytoestrogen supplements, a remarkable abnormal proliferative change of breast epithelial tissue with reddish and yellowish change under color mapping was shown (curve arrows); (a) estrogen therapy; (b) Chinese herb supplement; (c) Chinese herb (manly Chinese Angelica); (d) phytoestrogen supplement, probably benign small mass (white arrow) with normal yelloish-reddish on color mapping befor supplement.*

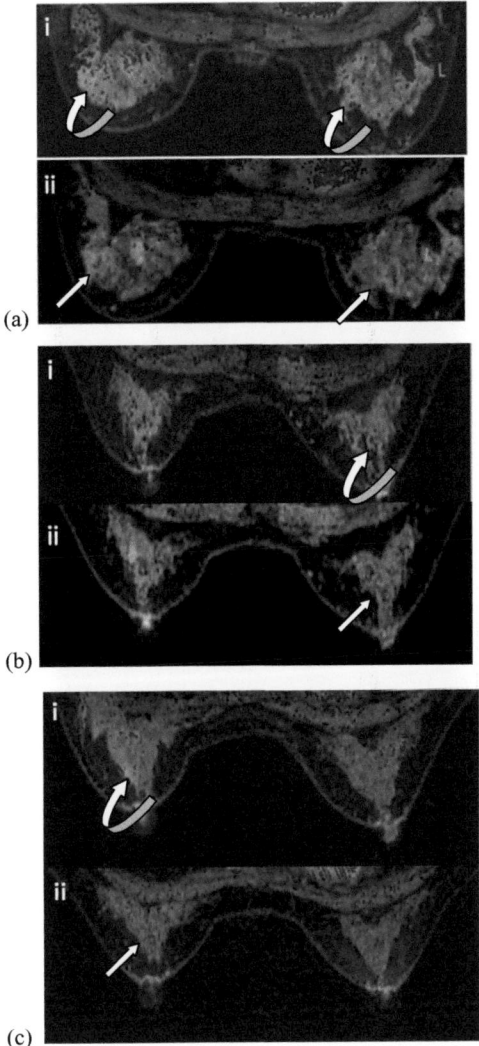

(a)

(b)

(c)

Figure 5a-5c . *(i) During estrogen therapy or phytoestrogen supplements, it shows diffusely proliferative change of bilateral breast epithelial tissue, represented by reddish and yellowish color parts on color mapping (curve arrows); (ii) after the drug and supplement cessation, MRI pictures show obvious improvement (straight arrows); (a) unknow dietary supplement (include Ganoderma lucidm); (b) royal*

jelly supplement; (c) hemical estrogen pills and royal jelly supplement.

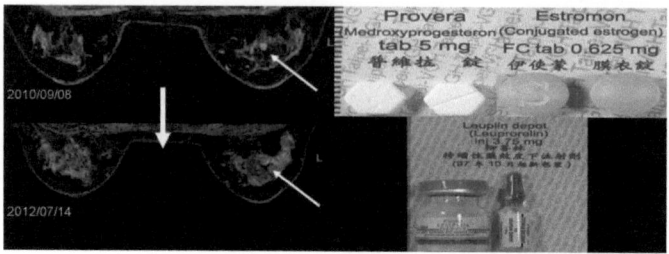

Figure 6 Before(left upper MRI image) and after(left lower MRI image) receiving

ovarian stimulation In Vitro Fertilization Protocols who using corresponding

medications and drug injection with estrogen and progesterone,there is significant

dvelopment of generalized of glandular tissue proliferation with increase yellow and

reddish color mapping. Particularly, interval progress change of a proliferative

mass(white arrows).

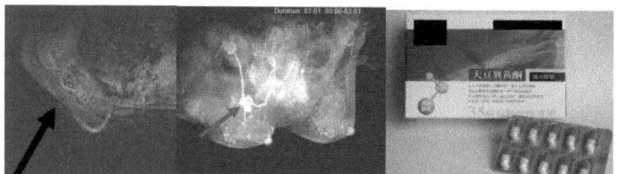

Figure 7 MRI images(left and middle) on a female patient with self palpated mass(red

arrow) with lymphatic node metastasis(black and red arrows), who was claimed to

have already received genistein(soybean extract) capsules(right) daily for 6

months.

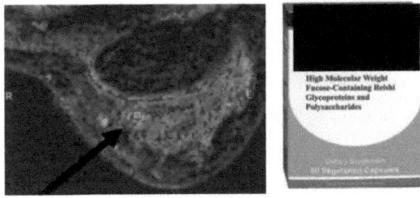

Figure 8 MRI image(left) on a female patient with malignant tumor in left breast,

found during health check up examination, who was claimed to have already

received Ganoderma lucidum extracted capsules(right) daily for 6 months.

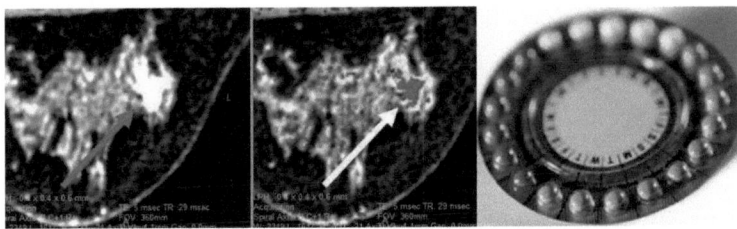

Figure 9 MRI images(left and middle) on a female patient with malignant tumor(red

and white arrows) in left breast, was found during her health check up examination.

She claimed to have already received combined estrogen and progesterone

treatment for dysmenorrheal problem over 22 years since 13 years old.

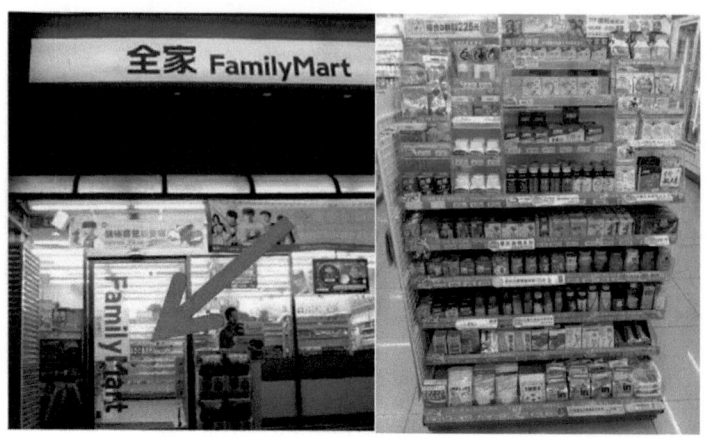

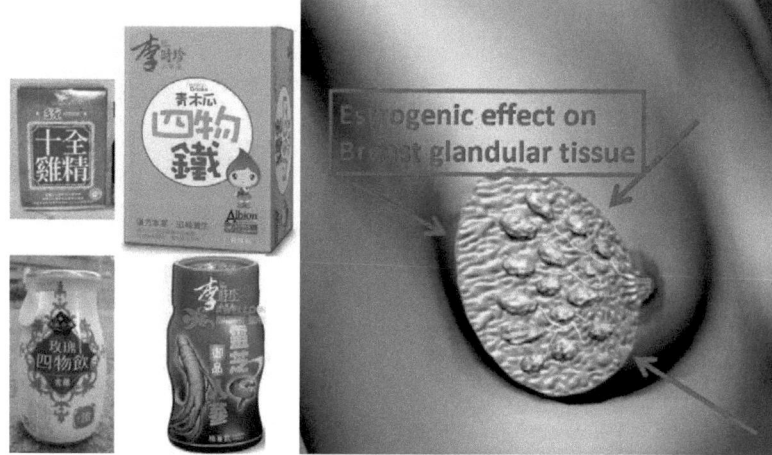

Figure 10 In Taiwan, many kinds of herb supplements(right upper and left lower) are

available for sales in convenient stores(left lower), with estrogenic effect on female

breast(right lower).

Molecular biology, Pathology and Breast MRI images

MRI provides a highly sensitive technique for early detection of abnormal breast

tissue. It is useful for identifying status of proliferation, angiogenesis, and

28

microvascular permeability, which may indicate early breast neoplasm formation.

We retrospectively studied 2795 breast MRI images from Taiwanese women and

classified them as either healthy or unhealthy according to BI-RADS categories. A

subgroup of our study patients had received estrogen supplements, containing

estrogen components or phytoestrogen, for at least 3 months. From our breast MRI

analysis, these two groups were compared and a significant difference was found

between them. The overuse of estrogen or phytoestrogen supplements can increase

breast glandular tissue proliferation, as reflected on MRI images. Such proliferation

may increase the patient's risk of future breast cancer. Therefore, we hypothesized

that phytoestrogen is involved in the breast tumorigenesis through activation of

proliferation and angiogenesis signaling. In the future, it is necessary to investigate

(a) the effect of phytoestrogen-induced proliferation and migration in-vitro and

in-vivo; (b) to study the effect of phytoestrogen-induced angiogenesis in endothelial

cells; and (c) to identify novel pathways or metabolomics related to

phytoestrogen-induced tumorigenic effects in breast cancer using protein

microarray analyses. The results of this study will provide important information on

the mechanism of breast tumorigenesis and may explain the persistent increasing

breast cancer incidence of Taiwanese young age women. (d) through the

mechanism, it help to discuss the method of prevention and treatment of breast cancer.

It is necessary to a better understanding of the tumor biology and microenvironment

characteristics related to different breast cancer subtypes and the extracellular

matrix composition assist in the prediction of biologic and therapeutic responses

improved treatment strategies and more individual patient management

Parameters of breast MRI

(1)Dynamic brMRI

Dynamic contrast-enhanced magnetic resonance imaging (Dynamic brMRI) is

capable to analysis on glandular tissue properties, such as vascular permeability,

contrast transfer coefficient (Ktrans), extracellular extravascular volume fraction(Ve)

and blood plasma volume fraction (Vp). It is useful for in vivo characterization of

tumor vasculature correlates with tumor type, histological grade, microvessel

density(MVD) , and biomarkers. Ktrans is the parameter for vessel perfusion and

permeability, while high Ktrans observed in the ER negative that may correlate to

the high MVD and high angiogenic activity. It also reflects less mature vessels with

incomplete vessel walls. Vp can be used as a tool for estimating vessel density. The

higher Vp found in the ER negative indicate a larger vascular space and higher

MVD in the basal-like tumors[74,75,76]. Ktrans is influenced by blood flow and

tumor vessel permeability, while the reduction in MVD increase in Ktrans is related to a change in vessel permeability rather than formation of new blood vessels. It was proposed that estrogen maintains VEGF expression enabling angiogenesis of breast tumor or abnormal breast glandular tissue. Aggressive tumors are known to have a high angiogenic activity, in order to maintain sufficient blood supply. Dynamic brMRI is useful on assessment of tumor vascularity, using gadodiamide(the contrast agent) enhancement depend on tissue perfusion and vessel permeability. Microvessel density(MVD) is a measure of angiogenesis in tissue sections, could be quantitatively demonstrated by dynamic brMRI. Besides, the endothelial cells and the vascular system regulated by a number of molecules such as vascular endothelial growth factors (VEGFs), which could be demonstrated by dynamic brMRI. VEGF is related to vascular endothelial cells, and responsible to proliferation and migration of cells, and forming new capillaries. VEGF was also known to augment capillary permeability. VEGF induced receptor phosphorylation is the crucial step lead to angiogenesis. It was also found that estradiol hormone receptor- positive luminal-like tumors of breast(ER positive) is related to phosphorylation of VEGF receptor. According to a in vivo MRI assessment on breast cancer xenografts study target on the histopathological microenvironment, ER positive was significant affected by available of estradiol on ER positive, but not affected on ER negative. On dynamic brMRI, cease supply of estradiol, tumors with ER positive cells had significant increase in median Ktrans and Ve. But no

significant change found in tumor with ER negative cells. [74,75,76] Thus,

dynamic brMRI can potentially differentiate between cancer subtypes and different

aggressiveness.

(2)MR spectroscopy(MRS)

MR spectroscopy(MRS) has demonstrated altered choline metabolism in malignant

breast cancer lesions. It has also been shown that elevation of the choline

metabolites phosphocholine (PC) and glycerophosphocholine (GPC) are associated

with malignant transformation of breast cancer cell lines. The genetic expression

profiles of the established tumor xenograft models represent the basal-like and

luminal A molecular subgroups of human breast cancer, and had significant

differences in choline metabolism pattern. According to previous MRS study, there

are found higher of creatine , choline Glycerophosphocholine, Glycine level of ER

negative breast cells than ER negative breast cells, but higher of Phosphocholine

and Taurine in ER positive negative breast cells[75,76].

(3)DWI and ADC

Diffusion weighted image(DWI) and the apparent diffusion coefficient (ADC) are the

most important parameter on water movement of water molecules in the tumor

microenvironment. ADC is calculated based on diffusion-weighted (DW) MRI data.

Malignant tumors have lower ADC values than normal tissue(figure11), include

higher cellularity, more disorganized tissue, and increased extracellular space

tortuosity. Benign is more likely to have higher ADC values, in verse

versa(figure12). It was found early increase in ADC of MRI measurement during

successful cancer therapies.

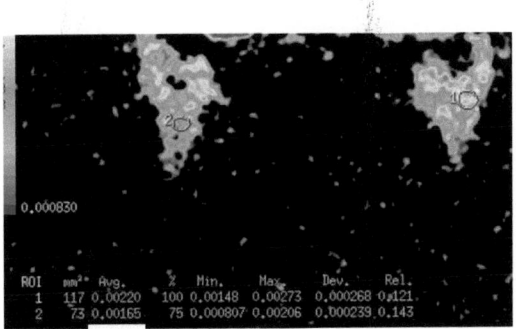

Figure11 : Precontrast Breast MRI analysis, with DWI and ADC mapping and

calculation(B valuve: 400), it shows reference point of normal left breast

tissue(Cursor 1) with ADC value: 2.20 (10-3 mm2/sec). On the contrast, the ROI on

right breast tumor(Cursor 2), with ADC value: 1.65(10-3 mm2/sec). The final

pathological result on the right breast tumor is invasive ductal carcinoma(lower

ADC value).

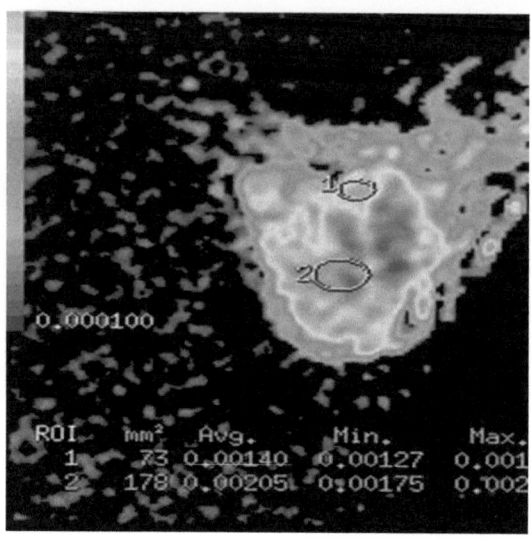

Figure12 :Precontrast Breast MRI analysis, with DWI and ADC mapping and

calculation(B valuve: 400), it shows reference point of normal left breast

tissue(Cursor 1) with ADC value: 1.40 (10-3 mm2/sec).On the contrast, the ROI on

right breast tumor(Cursor 2), with ADC value: 2.05(10-3 mm2/sec). The final

pathological result on the right breast tumor is fibrocystic change(higher ADC

value).

Low ADC is reflection of high cell density or an extracellular extravascular space

crammed with proteins. The low ADC values found in the luminal-like tumors are

in agreement with the high content of collagen and fibronectin in the stroma

Besides, increased ADC value is a result of increased extracellular diffusion due to cell shrinking or death. Tumor architecture and microenvironment change with

tumor progression or regression could be reflected on these MRI parameters[74].

On dynamic brMRI, cease supply of estradiol, tumors with ER positive cells had

significant increase in ADC[74].

Base on the previous studies, we summarized the corresponding MRI parameters on

breast tumors with ER positive and ER negative cells. Practically, breast MRI can

be used as a noninvasive tool for breast tumor characterization special attention to

angiogenesis and tumor microenvironment[74,75,76,77,78] (Table 2).

MRI measurement and related interpretations	Tumors with ER positive breast cells	Tumor with ER negative breast cells
MVD		Higher
Angiogenic activity		Higher
Vp		Higher
Ktrans, after cease supply of estradiol	Increase	
Ve, after cease supply of estradiol	Increase	
MRS: level of creatine		Increase
MRS: level of choline		Increase
MRS: level of Glycerophosphocholine		Increase
MRS: level of Glycine		Increase
MRS: level of Phosphocholine	Increase	
MRS: level of Taurine	Increase	
Median ADC values		Increase

Table 2 *Comparison of breast tumors with ER positive and ER negative subtypes on different MRI parameters*

Breast MRI also helps on the assessment of response after radiation therapy or during neo-adjuvant chemotherapy.

According to our clinical observation, magnetic resonance imaging (MRI) of the breast is extremely sensitive in detecting lesions and can identify the abnormal statuses of proliferation, angiogenesis, and microvascular permeability that occur in early breast neoplasm formation. In this study, we retrospectively reviewed breast MRI images of patients with a known estrogen and phytoestrogen intake to investigate a possible associated cancer risk. We used MRI results to assess the effect of estrogen and phytoestrogen on breast glandular tissue.

Over used of phytoestrogen and herb may responsible to increasing Taiwanese breast cancer incidence

It was found that women with low serum level of estrogen related to low incidence of breast cancer, on the contrary,high serum level estrogen corresponding to higher incidence of breast cancer [79,80]. Women in Taiwan, with increased dependency on Western diets that contains more fat and estrogen intake, is corresponding to earlier age of puberty, delayed arrival of menopause, and more obesity after menopause. Since estrogen is the major factor to promote proliferation of glandular cells ,thus, to increase the risk of breast cancer [80,81,82]. Past Study had been reported that dietary and nutritional factors accounted for about half of all cases of

breast cancer [81,82]. In the past, the tranditional Asian diet(rice and vegetable)

may help to reduce the incidence rate of breast cancer. But in Taiwan, this

advantage has disappeared, because the more use of the Western diet and nutrition.

Besides, it is also suspect the excessive use of traditional Chinese herbs or herbal

estrogen-like ingredient(phytoestrogens) may also contribute to the breast cancer

incidence[81,82].

As we know, women with proliferative breast disease has the risk of developing breast

cancer almost twice or higher possibility to the general female population.

Especially, to the women with atypical hyperplasia, even reported to have 5 times

risk taking than the normal female population. Women with family history of breast

cancer that combing atypical hyperplasia could be over 11 times of risk taking[83].

Many Chinese and Taiwanese women have been restrained from using ERT because

they were alerted of the risk of breast cancer. However, it is a common

misconception that plant-based food supplements (such as phytoestrogen) and

Chinese herbs assist postmenopausal women in avoiding breast cancer risks,

especially among Taiwanese women [84,85,86]. Furthermore, refraining from

estrogen, plant-based foods, and Chinese herb use does not guarantee that women

will be free from exogenous estrogen influences. Environmental estrogen pollution is also a factor because steroidal estrogen is constantly excreted into the environment. Pregnant women may excrete 10 μmol/d of estrogen, including estradiol and estrone. Chicken manure can contain more than 1 μmol/g of hormones (including estrogen), and other animals, such as cows, swine, horses, and goats, also excrete large amounts of estrogen. It is possible that environmental estrogen observed in water sources such as lakes and other water bodies can contaminate public drinking water supplies[87].

Many of our patients have told us that they believed that products from health food stores should be safe to use because they are "natural" or extracted from plants. However, hormone imbalances may be provoked by plants, health foods or herbs that mimic estrogen. Our clinical observations suggest that many young women begin to complain of sore or tender breasts and swelling before menstruation after they have started using dietary sup- plements that contain estrogen components or phytoestrogen. As far as we know, many herb drug has proved to process direct or indirect estrogenic effect, including herbal or Chinese herbs such as genistein, evening primrose oil, yam extract (yam extract), fungus, royal jelly, black cohosh, dong quai, motherwort, and different subgroups of Ginseng and so on.

Mammary cell membranes containing estrogen and progesterone receptors .

Approximately three-quarters of breast cancers are estrogen receptor (ER

-positive) , which means that estrogen causes the growth of these tumors .

However, the process of malignant transformation of breast cancer cells , not to

distinguish between patients with estrogen or by the patient intake of

phytoestrogens [88,89,90]. Synthetic estrogen (such as iso- estrogen xenoestrogen)

may take months to metabolism and excretion . The use of chemical and estrogen

has been found to increase the incidence of breast cancer has considerable

relevance . In contrast, the majority of food-grade supplemental estrogen or

phytoestrogen in vitro metabolism and discharged only a few days to a few weeks .

Therefore, short-term use of phytoestrogens may be connected with the incidence

of breast cancer is poor, but the long-term or excessive use of the same product may

not be safe. And although phytoestrogen supplement can reduce menopausal

symptoms, but may not prevent breast cancer[91,92,93].

In human breast cancer cell line study conducted shows that genistein inhibit and

stimulate cell proliferation. Found that genistein at low doses have mitogenic

effects at high doses have anti- proliferative effect. In a dose- dependent manner (in

a dose dependent manner), mouse breast cancer estrogen receptor -positive cell

lines (MCF-7 cells) first and then stimulated by growth inhibition of genistein, in

[88,89,90]. Study found that genistein imposed time, there will be different effects

on the breast. In addition , phytoestrogens genistein, may interfere with tamoxifen on breast cancer cell growth inhibition[94]. Should not be ignored genistein role in

promoting the potential of cancer[95]. In Asian countries, including China, Taiwan ,

Hong Kong and Singapore , many women seek natural herbal supplement or

conventional intake to relieve menopausal symptoms[91]. However, from a natural

or traditional Chinese medicine extracted phytoestrogens may stimulate breast

cancer cell line (MCF - 7) proliferation[95].Several studies have analyzed a variety

of herbal supplements and drugs. Cell cycle analysis showed that in MCF-7 cells

replicated with significant proliferative stimulus effects similar to human estrogen

(estradiol) [96,97,98,99]. Recalling this study breast MRI images show that

synthetic estrogen HRT and supplements containing ingredients are similar,

including Chinese herbal or plant estrogens . Nutritionists, naturopaths , Chinese

medicine practitioners , should pay attention to the excessive use of

estrogen-containing ingredients or plant estrogens or estrogen-like effects that

supplements issue. Such supplements can cause breast hyperplasia, and may

increase the risk of breast cancer. Family history or personal history of breast

cancer patients should be told to strictly avoid any type of estrogen or

phytoestrogen intake, unless it is unavoidable.

Tamoxifen and antiestrogen

According to our daily practice on breast MRI interpretation, some probably benign proliferative lesions that originally categorized as BIRADS 3, may transfer or not

transfer to malignancy. It is difficult to predict the exactly risk percentage of future

malignant transformation. Herein, we share our experiments with MRI images on

the before and after application of low dose tamoxifen on morphological change of

the benign proliferative lesions. Once we found tamoxifen can help to regress the

suspicious lesion, we keep observe the future change of that lesion. Thus, we have

found that tamoxifen is potentially a useful agent to help differentiate probably

benign lesion from high risk lesion in breast (figure13-16).

Applying tamoxifen on normal women with a risk of breast cancer has already been

advocated [100,101]. In January of 2013, The National Institute of Health and

Clinical Excellence of United Kingdom have launched a consultation on whether

tamoxifen could be given for up to five years. If approved later this year, the draft

guidelines would be the first of their kind in the United Kingdom. They also

announced that taking tamoxifen for five years could reduce high risk group with

family history of the disease. However, using tamoxifen to inhibit endogenous or

exogenous estrogen effects is occasionally difficult because of its potential side

effects. Since its introduction for clinical use in the early 1970s, synthetic

anti-estrogen tamoxifen citrate has been shown to contribute to controlling human

breast cancer and recurrence. Although its mechanisms of action and pharmacology are not completely understood, tamoxifen appears to act predominantly by blocking

the action of estrogen by binding to ERs. Clinical trials of tamoxifen for 1 to 2

years in primary breast cancer patients have shown consistent beneficial effects on

disease-free survival [98]. However, the gynecologic side effects of tamoxifen are

diverse and reflect the complexity of its mechanism of action; the most frequently

reported side effects are hot flashes. The most concerning gynecologic side effect is

endometrial disease in postmenopausal women[103]. Locally applying tamoxifen to

reduce the risk of breast glandular tissue damage caused by estrogen and

phytoestrogen is a concept that potentially reduces the dose-dependence systemic

effects of tamoxifen by minimizing its associated adverse effects.. In this study, we

focused on the efficacy of tamoxifen by examining the in vitro mammary glandular

cell-proliferative response to estrogen. Tamoxifen is an antagonist of the estrogen

receptor in breast tissue via its active metabolite, hydroxytamoxifen. In other

tissues such as the endometrium, it behaves as an agonist, and thus may be

characterized as a mixed agonist/antagonist. Tamoxifen is the usual endocrine

(anti-estrogen) therapy for hormone receptor-positive breast cancer in

pre-menopausal women, and is also a standard in post-menopausal women although

aromatase inhibitors are also frequently used in that

setting[104,105,106,107,108,109]. Some breast cancer cells require estrogen to grow. Estrogen binds to and activates the estrogen receptor in these cells.

Tamoxifen is metabolized into compounds that also bind to the estrogen receptor

but do not activate it. Because of this competitive antagonism, tamoxifen acts like a

key broken off in the lock that prevents any other key from being inserted,

preventing estrogen from binding to its receptor. Hence breast cancer cell growth is

blocked. Tamoxifen is currently used for the treatment of both early and advanced

ER+ (estrogen receptor positive) breast cancer in pre- and post-menopausal

women[104,105,106,107,108]. Additionally, it is the most common hormone

treatment for male breast cancer. It is also approved by the FDA for the prevention

of breast cancer in women at high risk of developing the disease.It has been further

approved for the reduction of contralateral (in the opposite breast)

cancer[104,105,106,107,108].

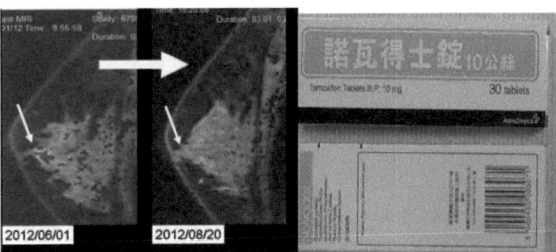

Figure13   Breast MRI images before(left) and after(middle) of a female patient who

was received Tamoxifen(daily dose:10mg) for over 2 and a half months for high

risk proliferative mass(white arrows) in right breast. The lesion was significant subsided.

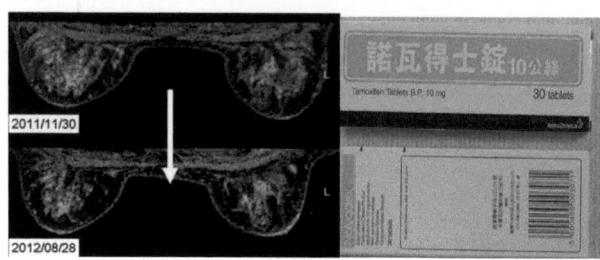

Figure14 Breast MRI images before(left upper) and after(left lower) of a female

patient who was received Tamoxifen(daily dose:10mg) for over 6 months for

proliferative breast glandular condition in bilateral breasts. The condition is

improved significantly.

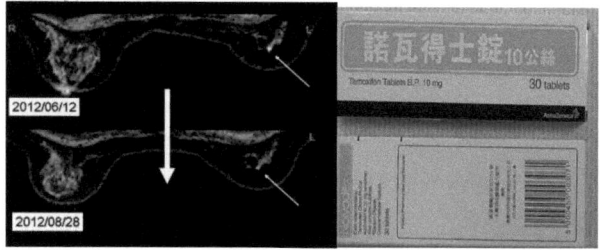

Figure15 Breast MRI images before(left upper) and after(left lower) of a female

patient who was received Tamoxifen(daily dose:10mg) for over 2 months for a low

risk probably benign proliferative fibroadenoma(white arrows) in left breast. The

lesion was found significant decreased in enhancement, reflecting decrease of proliferative change.

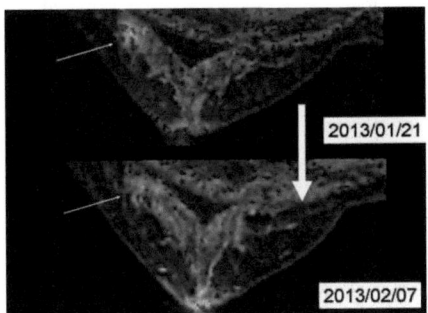

Figure16 Breast MRI images before(left upper) and after(left lower) of a female

patient who was received Tamoxifen(daily dose:10mg) for over 2 weaks a ill

defined lesion (white arrows) in lateral of right breast. The lesion was found

significant decreased in enhancement, reflecting regress change.

Correlation of MRI findings under effects of estrogen and tamoxifen with

biology and bio-molecular methods

(1)Cell proliferative change of MCF-10a under estrogen treatment and observed under

microscope (100X) and measured using colorimetric XTT

Colorimetric XTT assay is used as an indicator of cell proliferation, as determined by

its mitochondria-dependent reduction to formazone. Cells were plated at a density of 4 × 105 cells/well into 24-well plates for 24 h, treated with various

concentrations

of estrogen (0, 10, and 100 μM), and followed by a further zero to 3 d of treatment.

Cells were washed 3 times with PBS, and XTT (1 mg/ml) was added to the medium

for 3 h, and the supernatants were then collected. The absorbance was read at 450

nm using an enzyme-linked immunosorbent assay analyzer (ELISA, Gemini XPS

Molecular Devices, Sunnyvale, CA, USA).

(2)Results of Estrogen enhanced proliferation on MCF-10A: observed under

microscope(100X) and measured by colorimetric XTT(figure 17&18)

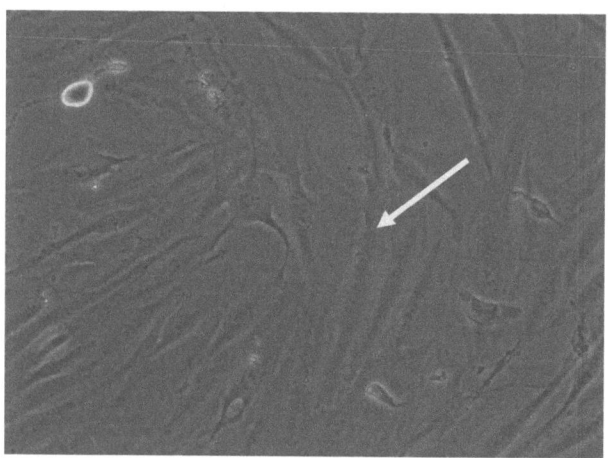

a

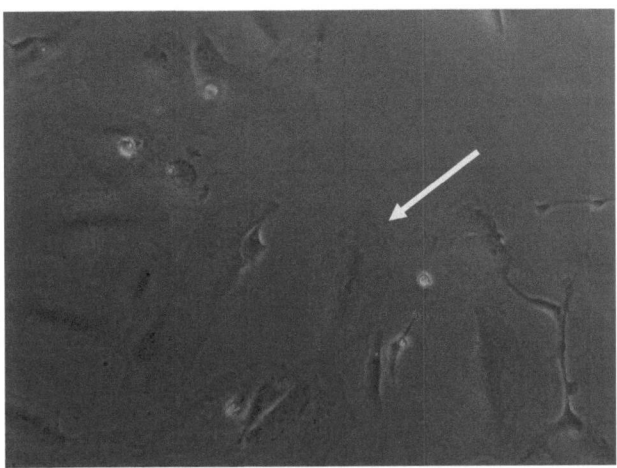

b

Figure17a&17b Effects of morphological changes of before(upper) and after(lower) induced by estrogen (on 100μmM) on breast normal cell line (MCF-10A)(white arrows)observing the morphology of cells under microscopy with a 100X power field.

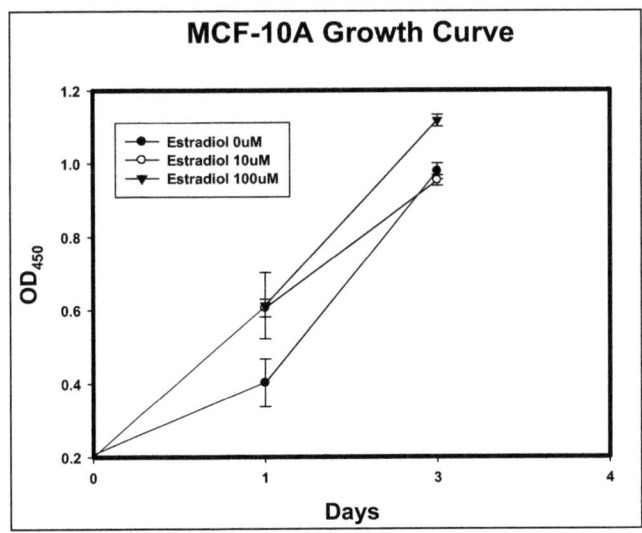

Figure 18 There are more significant proliferative change by 100μmM, compared to

both 0μmM and 10 μmM of estrogen doses.

<u>(3)Demonstration of Tamoxifen and phytonutrients concentration to inhibit cell</u>

<u>proliferation of MCF-10a under the effect of Estradiol</u>

According to the above method and the result of Estradiol concentration, to

demonstrate Tamoxifen concentration that capable to inhibit cell proliferation of

MCF-10a, by using colorimetric XTT assay as described above.

Tamoxifen (10 & 100 μ mole) is using to against estradiol concentrations of 100 μ

mole and 10 μ mole respectively(figure 19).

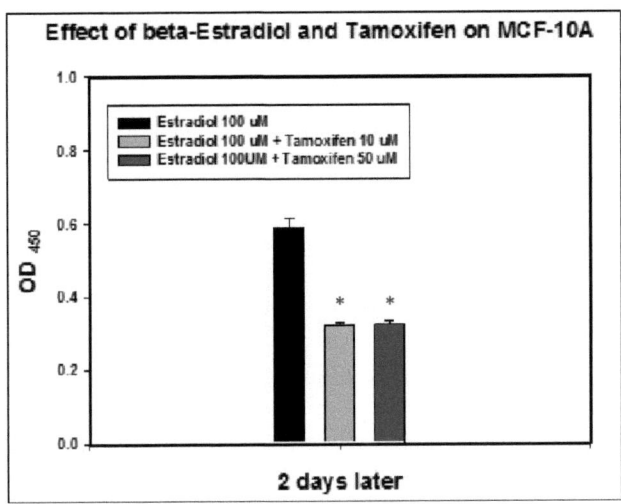

Figure19 By using 10 μ mole tamoxifen and 100 μ mole tamoxifen to inhibit proliferative stimulation of estrogen of 100 μ mole on MCF-10a.

Transdermal absorption of Tamoxifen

Tamoxifen is generally administered orally and parenterally. Tamoxifen undergo extensive hepatic metabolism after oral administration in people. Tamoxifen, despite being relatively effective when administered orally, particularly exhibits specific side effects such as appetite loss, abdominal cramps, nausea, and vomiting. Therefore, developing a therapeutic system to provide transdermal delivery is beneficial[109]. Previous research on tamoxifen has shown that no metabolic degradation of tamoxifen occurs in the skin; therefore, it is a suitable candidate(chemical) for transdermal delivery [110]. Tamoxifen has an elimination

49

half-life of 5 to 7 days, and its primary metabolite has an elimination half-life of 9

to 14 days. The metabolic and unchanged forms of tamoxifen can be obtained from

excretion [110]. Because this study demonstrated that tamoxifen can be

transdermally administered and accumulate subcutaneously over 10 days, it should

be evident that topical application provides a more effective distribution to breast

glandular tissue. It is recommended that the minimal dose of tamoxifen application

be employed to inhibit mammary epithelial cell proliferation when possible,

thereby reducing its side effects.

We believe that the application of tamoxifen as a transdermal treatment have

significant potential for preventing the estrogen-induced proliferative effect on

breast cells that result from estrogen and phytoestrogen supplement use, thereby

alleviating future breast cancer development and progression[111].

REFERENCES

1

Leung, T.K., Huang, P.J., Chen, C.S., Lin, Y.H., Wu, C.H. and Lee, C.M., Is breast MRI screening more
effective than digital mammography in Asian women? Journal of Experimental & Clinical Medicine
Volume 2, Issue 5 , Pages 245-250,(2010)

2

Ting-Kai Leung, Pai-Jung Huang, Chih-Hsiung Wu, Chi-Ming Lee, Chin-Sheng Hung, Hung-Hua
Liang, Jeng-Fong Chiou
Retrospective study of MRI images to examine the effects of estrogen supplementation on breast tissue:
A pilot study in Asian Taiwan, Health, Vol.5, No.7A4, 105-109 (2013)

3

Cancer Epidemiol Biomarkers Prev. 2005 Aug;14(8):1986-90.

Significant difference in the trends of female breast cancer incidence between Taiwanese and
   CaucasianAmericans: implications from age-period-cohort analysis.

Shen YC, Chang CJ, Hsu C, Cheng CC, Chiu CF, Cheng AL.

4

Shen, Y. C., Chang, C. J., Hsu, C., Cheng, C. C., Chiu, C. F. & Cheng, A. L. Significant
difference in the trends of female breast cancer incidence between Taiwanese and
Caucasian Americans: implications from age-period-cohort analysis. Cancer Epidemiol.
Biomarkers Prev. 14, 1986–1990 (2005).

5 Sim, X., Ali, R. A., Wedren, S., Goh, D. L., Tan, C. S., Reilly, M. et al. Ethnic differences
in the time trend of female breast cancer incidence: Singapore, 1968-2002. BMC
Cancer 6, 261 (2006).

6

Matsuno, R. K., Anderson, W. F., Yamamoto, S., Tsukuma, H., Pfeiffer, R. M.,
Kobayashi, K. et al. Early- and late-onset breast cancer types among women in the
United States and Japan. Cancer Epidemiol. Biomarkers Prev. 16, 1437–1442 (2007).

7

Kuo, W. H., Yen, A. M., Lee, P. H., Hou, M. F., Chen, S. C., Chen, K. M. et al. Incidence
and risk factors associated with bilateral breast cancer in area with early age diagnosis
but low incidence of primary breast cancer: analysis of 10-year longitudinal cohort in
Taiwan. Breast Cancer Res. Treat. 99, 221–228 (2006).

8

Kuo, W. H., Yen, A. M., Lee, P. H., Chen, K. M., Wang, J., Chang, K. J. et al. Cumulative
survival in early-onset unilateral and bilateral breast cancer: an analysis of 1907
Taiwanese women. Br. J. Cancer 100, 563–570 (2009).

9

Malone, K. E., Begg, C. B., Haile, R. W., Borg, A., Concannon, P., Tellhed, L. et al.
Population-based study of the risk of second primary contralateral breast
cancer associated with carrying a mutation in BRCA1 or BRCA2. J. Clin. Oncol. 28,
2404–2410 (2010).

10

Lynch, H. T., Silva, E., Snyder, C. & Lynch, J. F. Hereditary breast cancer: part I.

Diagnosing hereditary breast cancer syndromes. Breast J. 14, 3–13 (2008).

11

Kuo WH, Lin PH, Huang AC, Chien YH, Liu TP, Lu YS, Bai LY, Sargeant AM, Lin CH, Cheng
AL, Hsieh FJ, Hwu WL, Chang KJ.

J Hum Genet. 2012 Feb;57(2):130-8. doi: 10.1038/jhg.2011.142. Epub 2012 Jan 26.

Multimodel assessment of BRCA1 mutations in Taiwanese (ethnic Chinese) women with early-onset, b
ilateral orfamilial breast cancer.

12

Steven Shoei-Lung Li, H.-M. Tseng, Tsui-Ping Yang, Chia-Han Liu, Shiuh-Jen Teng, Hung-Wen Huang,
L.-M. Chen, Hsiao-Wei Kao, Jimmy H. Chen, Jau-Neng Tseng, Molecular characterization of
germline mutations in the BRCA1 and BRCA2 genes from breast cancer families in Taiwan

Human Genetics April 1999, Volume 104, Issue 3, pp 201-204

13

Cao W, Wang X, Gao Y, Yang H, Li JC. Anat Rec (Hoboken). 2013 Feb;296(2):273-8. doi:
10.1002/ar.22628. Epub 2012 Nov 23. BRCA1 germ-line mutations and tumor characteristics in
eastern Chinese women with familial breast cancer.

14

Seong MW, Cho S, Noh DY, Han W, Kim SW, Park CM, Park HW, Kim SY, Kim JY, Park SS.

Clin Genet. 2009 Aug;76(2):152-60. doi: 10.1111/j.1399-0004.2009.01202.x. Epub 2009 Jul 28.

Comprehensive mutational analysis of BRCA1/BRCA2 for Korean breast cancer patients: evidence of
a founder mutation.

15

Julian Peto, Nadine Collins, Rita Barfoot, Sheila Seal, William Warren, Nazneen Rahman, Douglas F.
Easton, Christopher Evans, Judith Deacon and Michael R. Stratton

J Natl Cancer Inst Volume 91, Issue 11Pp. 943-949.

Prevalence of BRCA1 and BRCA2 Gene Mutations in Patients With Early-Onset Breast Cancer

16

Hwei-Chung Wang, Chiu-Shong Liu, Chung-Hsing Wang, Ru-Yin Tsai,
Chia-Wen Tsai, Rou-Fen Wang, Chao-Hsiang Chang, Yueh-Sheng Chen,
Chang-Fang Chiu1, Da-Tian Bau, and Chih-Yang Huang

Chinese Journal of Physiology 53(2): 130-135, 2010

Significant Association of XPD Asp312Asn Polymorphism with Breast Cancer in Taiwanese Patients

17

Li, S. S., Tseng, H. M., Yang, T. P., Liu, C. H., Teng, S. J. & Huang, H. W. Molecular characterization of germline mutations in the BRCA1 and BRCA2 genes from breast cancer families in Taiwan. Hum. Genet. 104, 201–204 (1999).

18

Chen, S. T., Chen, R. A., Kuo, S. J. & Chien, Y. C. Mutational screening of breast cancer susceptibility gene 1 from early onset, bi-lateral, and familial breast cancer patients in Taiwan. Breast Cancer Res. Treat. 77, 133–143 (2003).

19

Chen, W., Pan, K., Ouyang, T., Li, J., Wang, T., Fan, Z. et al. BRCA1 germline mutations and tumor characteristics in Chinese women with familial or early-onset breast cancer. Breast Cancer Res. Treat. 117, 55–60 (2009).

20

Toh, G.T.K.P., Lee, S. S., Lee, D. S., Lee, S. Y., Selamat, S., Mohd, T. N. A. et al. BRCA1 and BRCA2 germline mutations in Malaysian women with early-onset breast cancer without a family history. PLoS ONE 3, e2024 (2008).

21

Ahn, S. H., Son, B. H., Yoon, K. S., Noh, D. Y., Han, W., Kim, S. W. et al. BRCA1 and BRCA2 germline mutations in Korean breast cancer patients at high risk of carrying mutations. Cancer Lett. 245, 90–95 (2007).

22

Liede, A. & Narod, S. A. Hereditary breast and ovarian cancer in Asia: genetic epidemiology of BRCA1 and BRCA2. Hum. Mutat. 20, 413–424 (2002).

23

Katalinic, A. and Rawal, R. (2008) Epidemiology decline in breast cancer incidence after decrease in utilisation of hormone replacement therapy. Breast Cancer Research Treatment, 107, 427-430. doi:10.1007/s10549-007-9566-z

24

Lupulescu A. Estrogen use and cancer incidence: a review. Cancer Invest

1995;13:287-95.

25

Henderson BE, Ross RK, Pike MC, Casagrande JT. Endogenous hormones as a major factor in human cancer. Cancer Res 1982;42:3232-9.

26

Pike MC, Spicer DV, Dahmoush L, Press MF. Estrogens, progestogens, normal breast cell proliferation, and breast cancer risk. Epidemiol Rev 1993;15:17-35.

27

Rosner B, Colditz GA. Nurses' Health Study: log-incidence mathematical model of breast cancer incidence. J Natl Cancer Inst 1996;88:359-64.

28.

Paffenbarger RS Jr, Kampert JB, Chang HG. Characteristics that predict risk of breast cancer before and after menopause. Am J Epidemiol 1980;112:258-68.

29

Clemons M, Goss P. N Engl J Med. 2001 Jan 25;344(4):276-85. Estrogen and the risk of breast cancer.

30

Zava DT, Dollbaum CM, Blen M.,Proc Soc Exp Biol Med. 1998 Mar;217(3):369-78. Estrogen and progestin bioactivity of foods, herbs, and spices.

31

Israel D, Youngkin EQ.,Pharmacotherapy. 1997 Sep-Oct;17(5):970-84. Herbal therapies for perimenopausal and menopausal complaints.

32

Alex Sparreboom, Michael C. Cox, Milin R. Acharya and William D. Figg, Herbal Remedies in the United States: Potential Adverse Interactions With Anticancer Agents Journal of Clinical Oncology June 15, 2004 vol. 22 no. 12 2489-2503

33

Hsieh, C.Y., Santell, R.C., Haslam, S.Z. and Helferich, W.G. (1998) Estrogenic effects of genistein on the growth of estrogen receptor-positive human breast cancer (MCF- 7) cells in vitro and in vivo. Cancer Research, 58, 3833- 3838.

34

Zava, D.T. and Duwe, G. (1997) Estrogenic and antiproli- ferative properties of genistein and other flavonoids in human breast cancer cells in vitro. Nutrition Cancer, 27, 31-40. doi:10.1080/01635589709514498

35

Wang, T.T., Sathyamoorthy, N. and Phang, J.M. (1996) Molecular effects of genistein on estrogen receptor medi- ated pathways. Carcinogenesis, 17, 271-275. doi:10.1093/carcin/17.2.271

36

Yager, J.D. and Davidson, N.E. (2006) Estrogen carcino- genesis in breast cancer. New England Journal of Medi- cine, 354, 270-282. doi:10.1056/NEJMra050776

37

Peeters, P.H.M., Keinan-Boker, L., van der Schouw, Y.T. and Grobbee, D.E. (2003) Phytoestrogens and breast can- cer risk: Review of the epidemiological evidence. Breast Cancer Research Treatment, 77, 171-183. doi:10.1023/A:1021381101632

38

Keinan-Boker, L., van der Schouw, Y.T., Grobbee, D.E. and Peeters, P.H.M. (2004) Dietary phytoestrogens and breast cancer risk. American Journal of Clinical Nutrition, 79, 282-288.

39

Hsieh, C.Y., Santell, R.C., Haslam, S.Z. and Helferich, W.G. (1998) Estrogenic effects of genistein on the growth of estrogen receptor-positive human breast cancer (MCF- 7) cells in vitro and in vivo. Cancer Research, 58, 3833- 3838.

40

Zava, D.T. and Duwe, G. (1997) Estrogenic and antiproli- ferative properties of genistein and other flavonoids in human breast cancer cells in vitro. Nutrition Cancer, 27, 31-40.

41

Wang, T.T., Sathyamoorthy, N. and Phang, J.M. (1996) Molecular effects of genistein on estrogen receptor medi- ated pathways. Carcinogenesis, 17, 271-275. doi:10.1093/carcin/17.2.271

42

Duffy, C., Perez, K. and Partridge, A. (2007) Implications of phytoestrogen intake for breast cancer. Ca-A Cancer Journal for Clinicians, 57, 260-277. doi:10.3322/CA.57.5.260

43

Bouker, K.B. and Hilakivi-Clarke, L. (2000) Genistein: Does it prevent or promote breast cancer? Environmental Health Perspectives, 108.

44

Yager, J.D. and Davidson, N.E. (2006) Estrogen carcino- genesis in breast cancer. New England Journal of Medi- cine, 354, 270-282. doi:10.1056/NEJMra050776

45

Mayo, J.L. (1997) A Natural approach to menopause. Clinical Nutrition Insights, 5, 1-8.

46

Huang, K.C. (1993) The pharmacology of Chinese herbs. CRC Press, Boca Raton.

47

Yapa, S.P., Shena, P., Lia, J., Leeb, L.S. and Yonga, E.L. (2007) Molecular and pharmacodynamic properties of es- trogenic extracts from the traditional Chinese medicinal herb, Epimedium. Journal of Ethnopharmacology, 113, 218-224. doi:10.1016/j.jep.2007.05.029

48

Wang, Z.Q. and Lou, Y.J. (2004) Proliferation-stimulating effects of icaritin and desmethylicaritin in MCF-7 cells. European Journal of Pharmacology, 504, 147-153. doi:10.1016/j.ejphar.2004.10.002

49

Lee Y, Jin Y, Lim W, Ji S, Choi S, Jang S, Lee S.
A ginsenoside-Rh1, a component of ginseng saponin, activates estrogen receptor in human breast carcinoma MCF-7 cells. J Steroid Biochem Mol Biol. 2003 Mar;84(4):463-8.

50

J.J. Michnovicz, Plant estrogens and human health, Ann. Surg. Oncol.

3 (1996) 513–514.

51

A.L. Murkies, G. Wilcox, S.R. Davis, Clinical review 92:
phytoestrogens, J. Clin. Endocrinol. Metabol. 83 (1998) 297–303.

52

Ivonne M. C. M. Rietjens, Ana M. Sotoca, Jacques Vervoort and Jochem Louisse
Mechanisms underlying the dualistic mode of action
of major soy isoflavones in relation to cell proliferation
and cancer risks
Mol. Nutr. Food Res. 2013, 57, 100–113

53

Hargreaves, D. F., Potten, C. S., Harding, C., Shaw, L. E.
et al., Two-week dietary soy supplementation has an estrogenic
effect on normal premenopausal breast. J. Clin.
Endocrinol. Metab. 1999, 84, 4017–4024.

54

Khan, S. A., Chatterton, R. T.,Michel, N., Bryk, M. et al., Soy
isoflavone supplementation for breast cancer risk reduction:
a randomized phase II trial. Cancer Prev. Res. (Phila).
2012, 5, 309–319.

55

National Toxicology Program (NTP), NTP technical report
on the toxicology and carcinogenesis study of genistein
(Cas No. 466-72-0) in Sprague-Dawley rats (feed
study). NTP TR 545 NIH publication No. 06-4430. Available
at http://ntp.niehs.nih.gov/ntp/about_ntp/BSC/TRRS/2006/
June/Board_Drafts/545_Web1.pdf.

56

Majid, S., Dar, A. A., Ahmad, A. E., Hirata, H. et al., BTG3
tumor suppressor gene promoter demethylation, histone
modification and cell cycle arrest by genistein in renal cancer.
Carcinogenesis 2009, 30, 662–670.

57

Majid, S., Dar, A. A., Shahryari, V., Hirata, H. et al., Genistein
reverses hypermethylation and induces active histone
modifications in tumor suppressor gene B-cell translocation
gene 3 in prostate cancer. Cancer 2010, 116, 66–76.

58

Day, J. K., Bauer, A. M., desBordes, C., Zhuang, Y. et al.,
Genistein altersmethylation patterns in mice. J. Nutr. 2002,
132, 2419S–2423S.

59

Zhang, Q.-X., Hilsenbeck, S. G., Fuqua, S. A. W., Borg,
A ., Multiple splicing variants of the estrogen receptor are
present in individual human breast tumors. J. Steroid
Biochem. Mol. Biol. 1996, 59, 251–260.

60

Lu, B., Leygue, E., Dotzlaw, H.,Murphy, L. J. et al., Estrogen
receptor-_ mRNA variants in human and murine tissues.
Mol. Cell. Endocrinol. 1998, 138, 199–203.

61

Davies, M. P. A., O'Neill, P. A., Innes, H., Sibson, D. R. et al.,
Correlation of mRNA for oestrogen receptor beta splice
variants ER_1, ER_2/ER_cx and ER_5 with outcome in
endocrine-treated breast cancer. J. Mol. Endocrinol. 2004,
33, 773–782.

62

Auboeuf, D., Batsche, E., Dutertre, M., Muchardt, C. et al.,
Coregulators: transducing signal from transcription to alternative
splicing. Trends Endocrinol. Metab. 2007, 18,
122–129.

63

Sotoca, A.M., Vervoort, J., Rietjens, I. M. C. M., Gustafsson,
J-A° ., Human ER_ and ER_ splice variants: understanding
their domain structure in relation to their biological roles in
breast cancer cell proliferation. Biochemistry, 2012, Chapter
5, pp 141–160.

64

Cho J, Park W, Lee S, Ahn W, Lee Y.
J Clin Endocrinol Metab. 2004 Jul;89(7):3510-5.
Ginsenoside-Rb1 from Panax ginseng C.A. Meyer activates estrogen receptor-alpha and -beta,
    independent of ligand binding.

65

Lee YJ, Jin YR, Lim WC, Park WK, Cho JY, Jang S, Lee SK.
Ginsenoside-Rb1 acts as a weak phytoestrogen in MCF-7 human breast cancer cells.
Arch Pharm Res. 2003 Jan;26(1):58-63.

66

ISABELLE DUMAS1 and CAROLINE DIORIO
ANTICANCER RESEARCH 31: 4369-4386 (2011)
Estrogen Pathway Polymorphisms and Mammographic Density

67

Elisabeth Couto, Samera Azeem Qureshi,Solveig Hofvind , Marit Hilsen, Hildegunn Aase,
Per Skaane , Lars Vatten , Giske Ursin
Breast Cancer Res Treat (2012) 132:297–305
Hormone therapy use and mammographic density
in postmenopausal Norwegian women

68

Erguvan-Dogan B, Whitman GJ, Kushwaha AC, Phelps MJ, Dempsey PJ. BI-RADS-MRI: a primer.
    Am J Roentgenol 2006;187:W152–60.

69

TW Stephens. Illustrated Breast Imaging Reporting and Data System (BI-RADS). 3rd ed. Reston, Va.:
    American College of Radiology, 1998.

70

Liberman L, Menell JH. Breast Imaging Reporting and Data System (BI-RADS). *Radiol Clin N Am* 2002;40:409–30.

71

Leung TK, Chu JS, Huang PJ, Lee CM, Lin YH, Chen CS, Tai CJ, Wu CH. Breast MRI for Monitoring Images of an 'Adenomyoepithelioma with Malignant Features', Before, During, and After Chemotherapy. *Breast J* 2010;16:652–3.

72

Leung TK, Huang PJ, Lee CM, Chen CS, Wu CH, Chao JS. Can breast magnetic resonance imaging demonstrate characteristic findings of preoperative ductal carcinoma in situ in Taiwanese women? *Asian J Surg* 2010;33:143–9.

73

Leung TK, Huang PJ, Lee CM, Chen CS. Silicone Breast implant with intracapsular rupture coexisting with locally advanced carcinoma. *Breast J* 2012; 18:76–7.

74

Huuse EM, Moestue SA, Lindholm EM, Bathen TF, Nalwoga H, Krüger K, Bofin A, Maelandsmo GM, Akslen LA, Engebraaten O, Gribbestad IS.,*J Magn Reson Imaging. 2012 May;35(5):1098-107. doi: 10.1002/jmri.23507. Epub 2011 Dec 14.*

In vivo MRI and histopathological assessment of tumor microenvironment in luminal-like and basal-like breast cancer xenografts.

75

S. A. Moestue, E. M. Huuse, O. Engebraten, B. Sitter, G. M. Mælandsmo, T. F. Bathen1, and I. S. Gribbestad, Proc. Intl. Soc. Mag. Reson. Med. 17 (2009)

Choline metabolic composition correlates to basal-like and luminal A genetic subtypes in orthotopic breast cancer xenografts

76

Anna Bergamaschi, Geir Olav Hjortland, Tiziana Triulzi, Therese Sorlie,

Hilde Johnsen, Anne Hansen Ree, Hege Giercksky Russnes, Sigurd Tronnes,

Gunhild M. Maelandsmo, Oystein Fodstad, Anne-Lise Borresen-Dale,

Olav Engebraaten, Molecular profiling and characterization of luminal-like and basal-like in vivo breast cancer xenograft models

Molecular Oncology 3 (2009) 469–482

77

Laura Martincich, Veronica Deantoni, Ilaria Bertotto, Stefania Redana, Franziska Kubatzki, Ivana
  Sarotto, Valentina Rossi, Michele Liotti, Riccardo Ponzone, Massimo Aglietta,
European Radiology July 2012, Volume 22, Issue 7, pp 1519-1528
Correlations between diffusion-weighted imaging and breast cancer biomarkers

78

Raphael Richard, Isabelle Thomassin, Marion Chapellier, Aurélie Scemama, Patricia de Cremoux,
  Mariana Varna, Sylvie Giacchetti, Marc Espié, Eric de Kerviler, Cedric de Bazelaire,
Diffusion-weighted MRI in pretreatment prediction of response to neoadjuvant chemotherapy in
  patients with breast cancer, European Radiology September 2013, Volume 23, Issue 9, pp 2420-2431

79

Key TJ, Chen J, Wang DY, Pike MC, Boreham J. Sex hormones in women in rural China and in Britain.
  Brit J Cancer 1990;62:631–6.

80

Clemons M, Goss P. Estrogen and the Risk of Breast Cancer. *New Engl J Med* 2001;344:276–85.

81

Tsai AC, Liou JC, Chang MC, Chuang YL. Influence of diet and physical activity on aging-associated
  body fatness and anthropometric changes in older Taiwanese. *Nutr Res* 2007;27:245–51.

82

Hsieh SC, Lai JN, Lee CF, Hu FC, Tseng WL, Wang JD. The prescribing of Chinese herbal products in
  Taiwan: a cross-sectional analysis of the national health insurance reimbursement database.
  Pharmacoepidemiol Drug Saf 2008;17:609–19.

83

Dupont WD, Page DL. Risk Factors for Breast Cancer in Women with Proliferative Breast Disease.
  New Engl J Med 1985;312:146–51.

84

Hsieh, C.Y., Santell, R.C., Haslam, S.Z., Helferich, W.G., 1998. Estrogenic effects of genistein on the
  growth of estrogen receptor-positive human breast cancer (MCF-7) cells in vitro and in vivo. Cancer
  Res. 58, 3833-3838.

85

Hsieh, S.C., Lai, J.N., Lee, C.F., Hu, F.C., Tseng, W.L., Wang, J.D., 2008. The prescribing of Chinese herbal products in Taiwan: a cross-sectional analysis of the national health insurance reimbursement database. Pharmacoepidemiol Drug Saf. 17, 609-619.

86

Zava, D.T., Duwe, G., 1997. Estrogenic and antiproliferative properties of genistein and other flavonoids in human breast cancer cells in vitro. Nutr Cancer. 27, 31-40.

87

Barel-Cohen, K., Shore, L.S., Shemesh, M., Wenzel, A., Mueller, J., Kronfeld-Schor, N., 2006. Monitoring of natural and synthetic hormones in a polluted river. J Environ Manage. 78, 16-23.

88

Hsieh CY, Santell RC, Haslam SZ, Helferich WG. Estrogenic effects of genistein on the growth of estrogen receptor-positive human breast cancer (MCF-7) cells in vitro and in vivo. *Cancer Res* 1998;58:3833–8.

89

Zava DT, Duwe G. Estrogenic and antiproliferative properties of genistein and other flavonoids in human breast cancer cells in vitro. *Nutr Cancer* 1997;27:31–40.

90

Wang TT, Sathyamoorthy N, Phang JM. Molecular effects of genistein on estrogen receptor mediated pathways. *Carcinogenesis* 1996;17:271–5.

91

Yager JD, Davidson NE. Estrogen Carcinogenesis in Breast Cancer. *New Engl J Med* 2006;354:270–82.

92

Peeters PHM, Keinan-Boker L, van der Schouw YT, Grobbee DE. Phytoestrogens and breast cancer risk: Review of the epidemiological evidence. B*reast Cancer Res Tr* 2003;77:171–83.

93.

Keinan-Boker L, van der Schouw YT, Grobbee DE, Peeters PHM. Dietary phytoestrogens and breast cancer risk. *Am J Clin Nutr* 2004;79:282–8.

94

Duffy C, Perez K, Partridge A. implications of phytoestrogen intake for breast cancer. *Ca-Cancer J Clin* 2007;57:260–77.

95

Bouker KB, Hilakivi-Clarke L. Genistein: does it prevent or promote breast cancer? *Environ Health Persp* 2000;108.

96

Mayo JL. A Natural Approach to Menopause. Clin Nutr Insights 1997;5:1–8.
m23. Huang KC. *The Pharmacology of Chinese Herbs*. Boca Raton, FL: CRC Press, 1993.

97

Yapa SP, Shena P, Lia J, Leeb LS, Yonga EL. Molecular and pharmacodynamic properties of estrogenic extracts from the traditional Chinese medicinal herb, Epimedium. *J Ethnopharmacol* 2007;113:218–24.

98

Wang ZQ, Lou YJ. Proliferation-stimulating effects of icaritin and desmethylicaritin in MCF-7 cells. *Eur J Pharmacol* 2004;504:147–53.

99

Åberg UW, Saarinen N, Abrahamsson A, *et al*. Tamoxifen and flaxseed alter angiogenesis regulators in normal human breast tissue in vivo. *PLoS One* 2011;6:e25720.

100

Sakata M, Ikeda T, Imoto S, *et al*. Prevention of mammary carcinogenesis in C3H/OuJ mice by green tea and tamoxifen. *Asian Pac J Cancer Prev* 2011;12:567–71.

101

Love RR. Tamoxifen therapy in primary breast cancer: biology, efficacy, and side effects. *J Clin Oncol* 1989;7:803–15.

102

Katalinic A, Rawal R. Epidemiology- Decline in breast cancer incidence after decrease in utilisation of hormone replacement therapy. *Breast Cancer Res Tr* 2008;107:427–30.

103

Kisanga ER, Mellgren G, Lien EA. Anticancer Res. 2005 Nov-Dec;25(6C):4487-92.

Excretion of hydroxylated metabolites of tamoxifen in human bile and urine.

104

Coezy E, Borgna JL, Rochefort H. Cancer Res. 1982 Jan;42(1):317-23.

Tamoxifen and metabolites in MCF7 cells: correlation between binding to estrogen receptor and
inhibition of cell growth.

105

Allred DC, Anderson SJ, Paik S, Wickerham DL, Nagtegaal ID, Swain SM, Mamounas EP, Julian TB,
Geyer CE Jr, Costantino JP, Land SR, Wolmark N. J Clin Oncol. 2012 Apr 20;30(12):1268-73. doi:
10.1200/JCO.2010.34.0141. Epub 2012 Mar 5.

Adjuvant tamoxifen reduces subsequent breast cancer in women with estrogen receptor-positive ductal
carcinoma in situ: a study based on NSABP protocol B-24.

106

Charlie Schmidt, The Breast Cancer Chemoprevention Debate
JNCI Vol. 103, Issue 22 | November 16, 2011

107

Sakata M, Ikeda T, Imoto S, Jinno H, Kitagawa Y. Asian Pac J Cancer Prev. 2011;12(2):567-71.
Prevention of mammary carcinogenesis in C3H/OuJ mice by green tea and tamoxifen.

108

Åberg UW, Saarinen N, Abrahamsson A, Nurmi T, Engblom S, Dabrosin C.
Tamoxifen and flaxseed alter angiogenesis regulators in normal human breast tissue in vivo.
PLoS One. 2011;6(9):e25720.

109

Pathan IB, Setty CM. Enhancement of transdermal delivery of tamoxifen citrate using nanoemulsion
vehicle. *Int J Pharm Tech Res* 2011;3:287–97.

110

Zhao K, Singh S, Singh J. Effect of menthone on the in vitro percutaneous absorption of tamoxifen and
skin reversibility. *Int J Pharm* 2010;219:177–81.

111

Ting Kai Leung ,Patent Application(No.101129868), Republic of China(Taiwan), Topical used formula of anti-estrogen. (2012).

Authors' Information

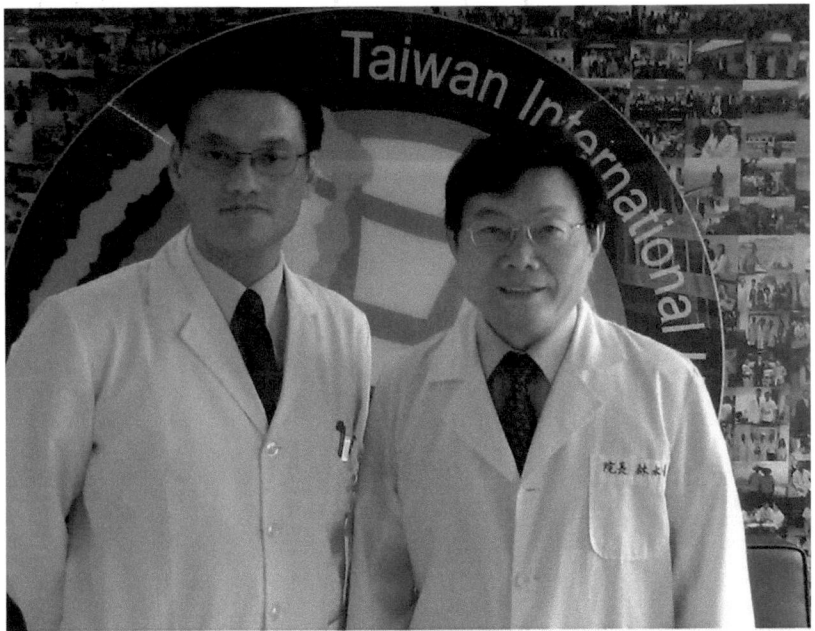

(1)Author Name: **Dr. Ting-Kai Leung, MD (left)**

Specialty Experience: Internal Medicine Resident and Radiologist (Department

Director)

Academic positions: Ass. Professor on 'medical physics' and 'clinical radiology' for

Taipei Medical and Fu Jen Catholic Universities. Since 2005, invite as Quality

Assurance Committee of National Health Authority Breast Screening in Taiwan.

Corresponding investigator for a Global Human Trial center: Godovist (BAYER)

for Breast MRI

Related Publications:

Contributing Writer for China Times newspaper column - (Kyorin fax) and (Hua

Tuo fax); Academic publications in over hundred in numbers, include ten research

articles on breast related topics. Besides, written a book chapter: "The Application

of Breast MRI on Asian Women (Dense Breast Pattern)", published in the book of

"Imaging of the Breast - Technical Aspects and Clinical Implication"(Edited by:

Laszlo Tabar).

(2)Author Name: **Dr.Shoei-Loong Lin, MD (right)**

Clinical Professor of Surgery in Taipei Medical University and National Yang Ming

University, as well as superintendent of National Taipei Hospital of Ministry of

Health and Welfare in Taiwan. He is one of the most experienced breast surgeons in

Taiwan and was the first clinician who recommends the benefit of breast MRI for

early breast cancer diagnosis.

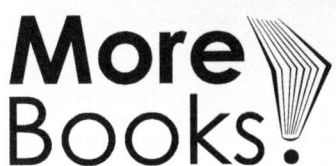
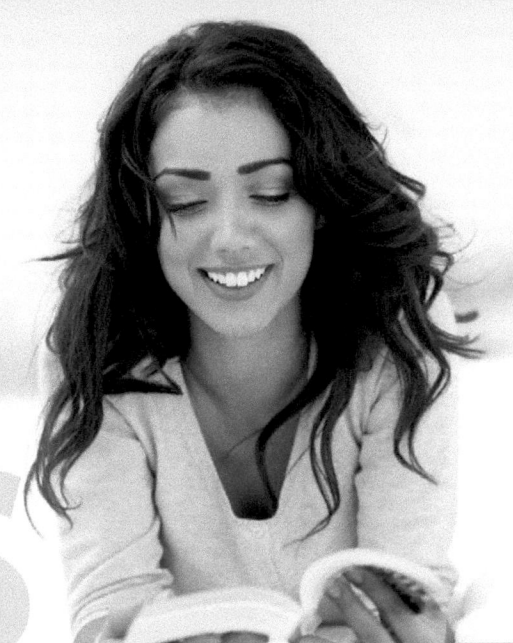
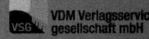